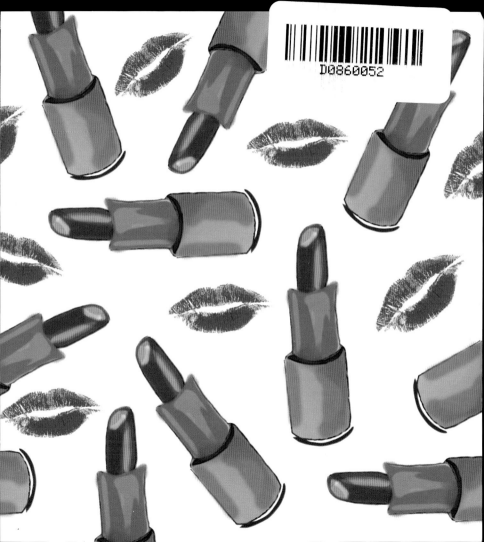

D0860052

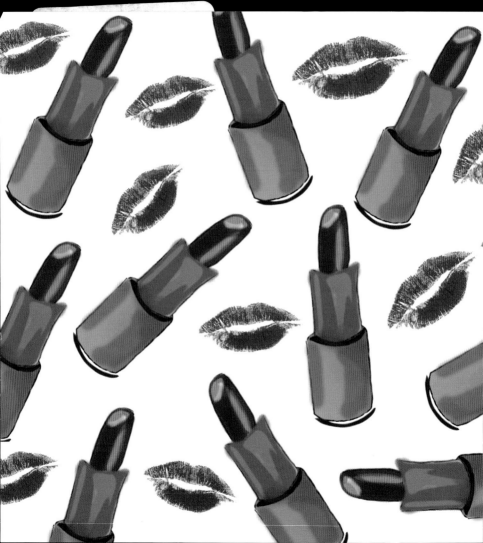

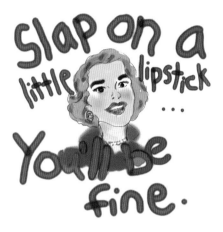

Slap on a little lipstick ... You'll be fine.

jodi hills

TRISTAN Publishing
Minneapolis

To every girl, in any shade, who stands in front
of that mirror and sees all the possibilities that lie within.
Thanks, Mom, for giving me the courage to look.

jodi hills

Library of Congress Cataloging-in-Publication Data

Hills, Jodi, 1968-
Slap on a little lipstick--you'll be fine / Jodi Hills.
 p. cm.
ISBN 0-931674-74-3 (alk. paper)
1. Women--Psychology--Miscellanea. 2. Resilience (Personality trait)--
    Miscellanea. 3. Feminine beauty (Aesthetics)--Miscellanea. I. Title.

HQ1206.H5184 2005
646.7'042--dc22

                                                    2005055984

TRISTAN Publishing, Inc.
2300 Louisiana Avenue North, Suite B
Golden Valley, MN 55427
www.tristanpublishing.com

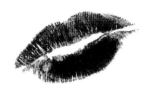

Is it
shallow...

or simply brilliant,

that we've figured out
survival can be

a beautiful thing...

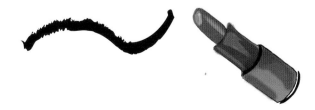

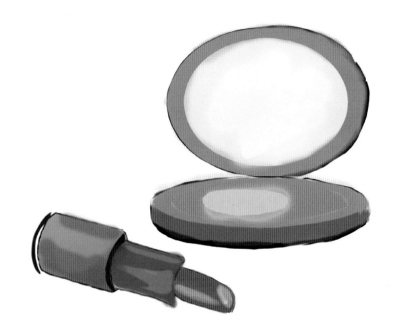

We've figured out that we can
stand in front of that mirror,
uncertain of what
the day may bring...

Stand in front of that mirror
with five pounds to lose,
overworked,
underpaid,

single, married,

tall, short,

wanting, waiting...

and

look at life

with a different hue.

We stand in front of
that mirror
and pull out a tube of
Mocha Pink,
Alfresco Brick,
or Ruby Rose...

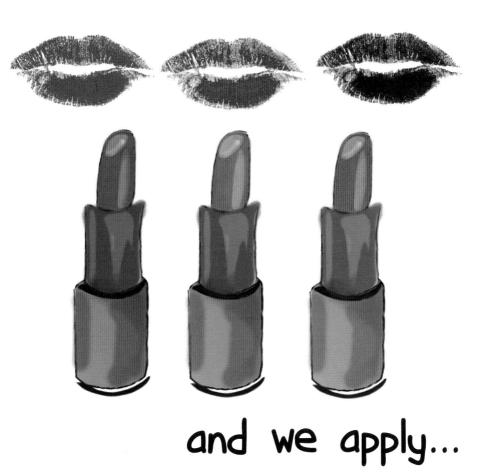

and we apply...

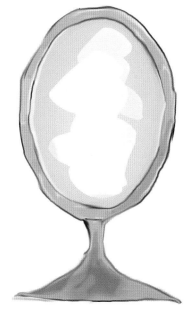

confident

Confident that whatever lies ahead...
bosses,
children,
cramps,
deadlines,
decisions,
hellos and good-byes...

we stand **a bit more secure**
in ourselves,
believing the words
our mothers spoke before us...

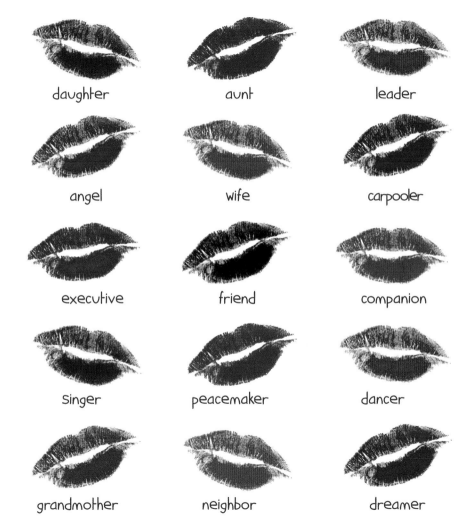

daughter

aunt

leader

angel

wife

carpooler

executive

friend

companion

singer

peacemaker

dancer

grandmother

neighbor

dreamer

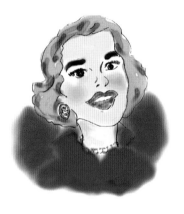

"Slap on a little lipstick, you'll be fine."

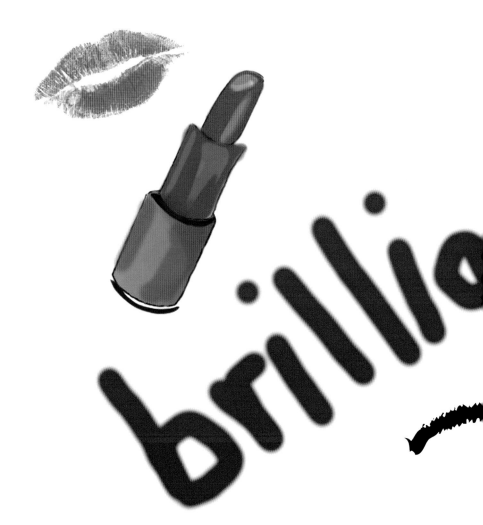

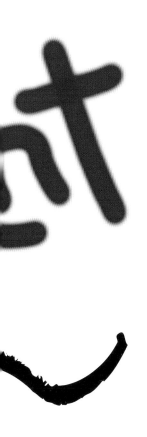

So I say to you
that it *is* **brilliant**...
and if it's a
smidge shallow,
does that
really
hurt anyone

?

What is the harm
in feeling good about yourself...
presenting yourself to the world
with lip-lined confidence ?

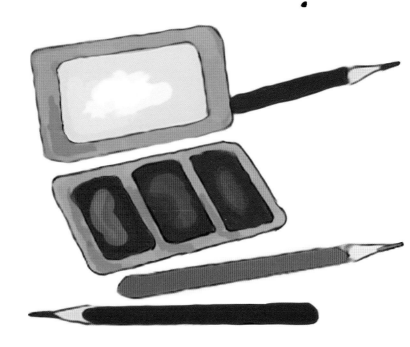

If your brightened lips
brighten your possibilities,
and lighten your load just a little,
then I say

apply!

apply!

apply!

This is not to discredit
the support systems around us.

Nothing can replace
the power of love,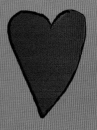

or a good personal trainer...

And I certainly won't argue
the value of intelligence,

or the quick fix of a
fine piece of chocolate,

but these are not always
available...

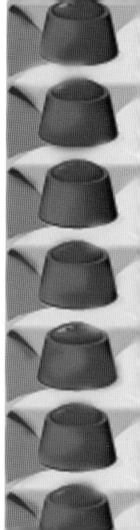

Good psychiatrists are hard to find,
and rarely fit inside
the zip pocket of your
favorite clutch,
like my
Apricot
Beige #7.

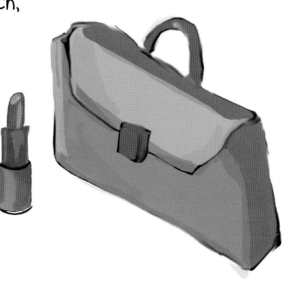

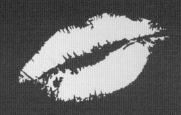

The world is both physically
and emotionally demanding...
enough to drain the color
out of the strongest faces.

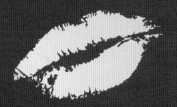

Roles are changing faster
than fashion trends,

but constant can be our belief
in ourselves and each other.

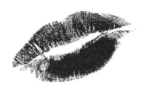

believer

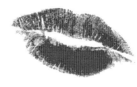

provider

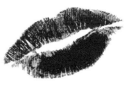

protector

Constant can be
our smiles in the mirror,
or the simple words
shared with a friend -
"that's a great color on you."

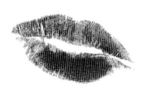

designer

inventor

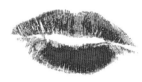

comforter

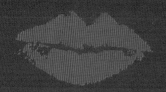

Sure it's simple
to slap on a little lipstick –

but does everything
have to be so hard?

Give yourself a break.

Take the time to enjoy that glorious sunrise,

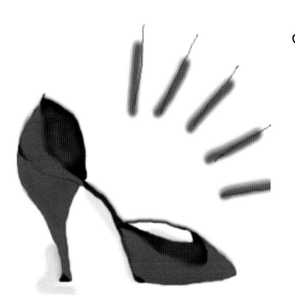

or the feel of Italian leather shoes against your feet, and the way they make your calves look smaller.

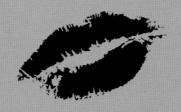

Even if it just gives you an escape
for a few moments...

find the
beauty.

It's never wrong
to try and be happy...

to feel beautiful
inside and out.

happy happy happy

Yes, it's true it's not all about outer beauty...
inner beauty is definitely
more than important...

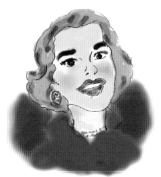
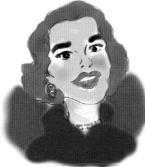
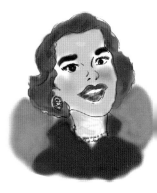

nobody likes a mean girl,
in any shade!

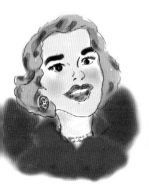
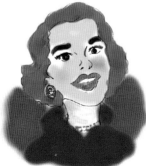
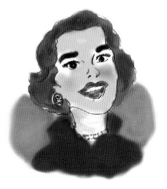

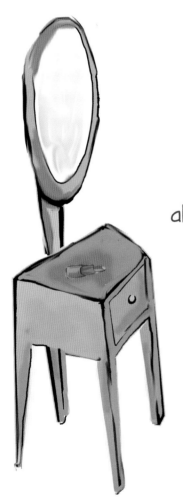

Now, we probably
won't solve
all the world's problems
by slapping on a
little lipstick,

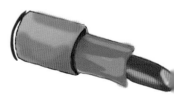

but in altering a few attitudes,
and brightening a few spirits,
who's to say
that we won't
change things,

for the better.

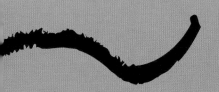

So even on your clouded days,

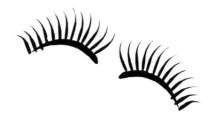

remember, no one wears Rich'n Rosy

quite like you...

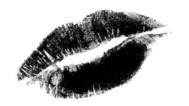

No one smiles behind a Passionate Pink

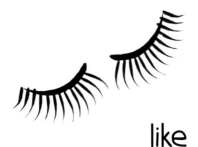

like you...

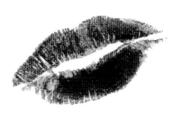

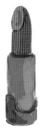

You are this day's survivor
and a thing of beauty.

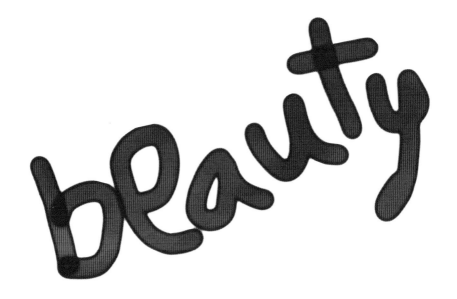

You can stand in front
of any crowd,
or any mirror,
and feel good about yourself.

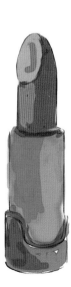

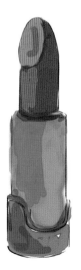

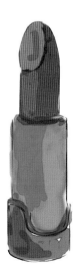

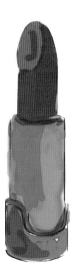

Whether you

are a

💋 daughter, or

💋 mother, or

💋 sister, or

💋 girlfriend,

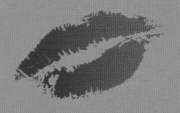

you are proof positive
that daily survival can be
a beautiful thing!

No matter what
this world throws at you,
you will thrive,
believing in mother's
simply brilliant words,

"Slap on a little lipstick, you'll be fine."

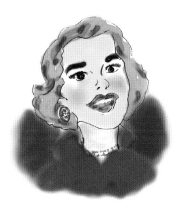

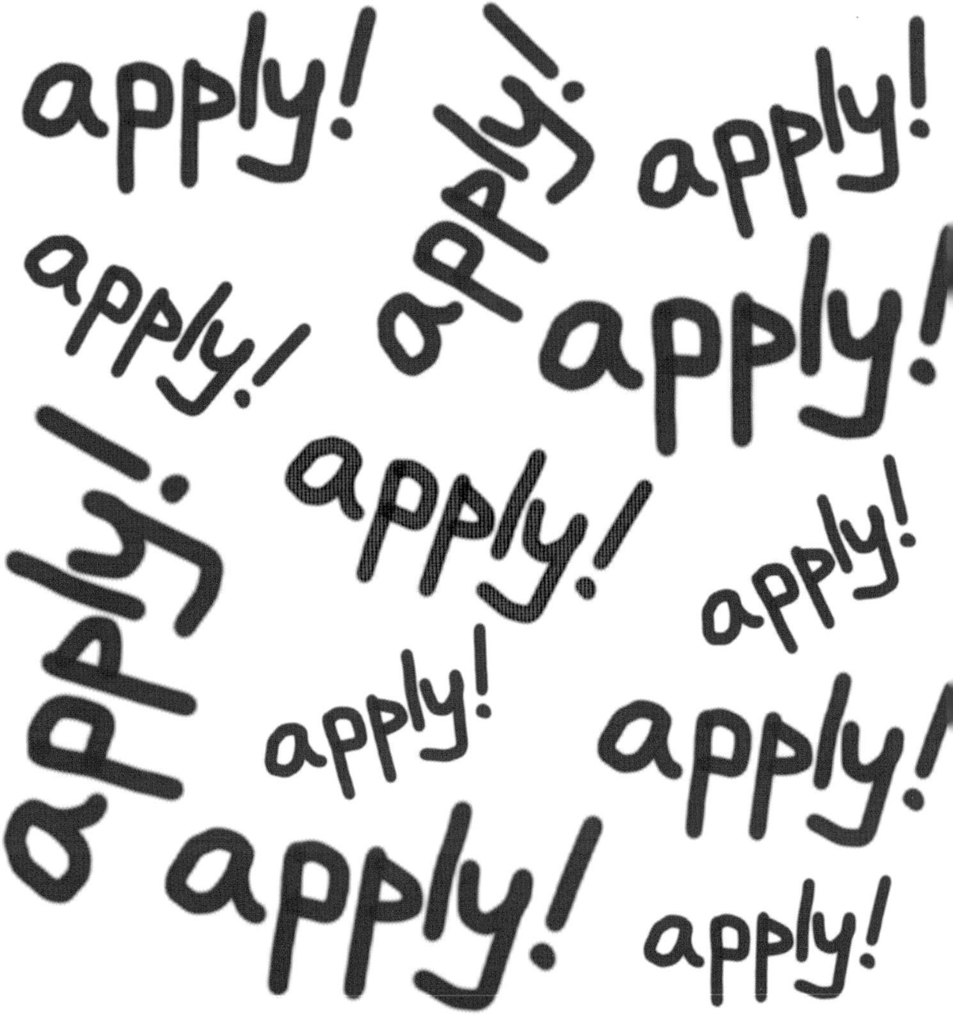

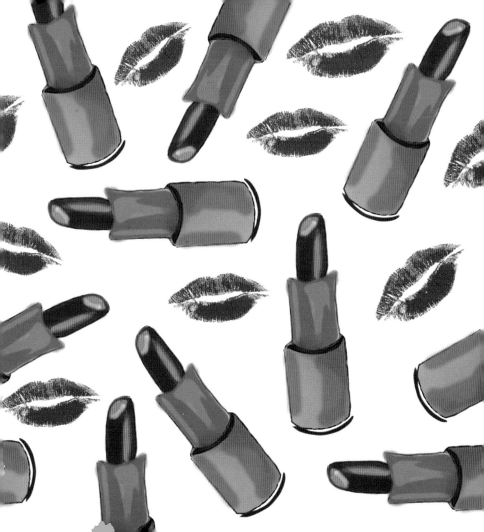

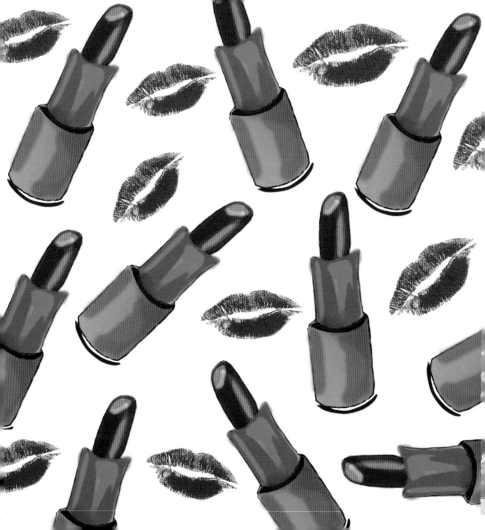